MW01242326

Contents

1

Introduction

The Volumetric Diet emphasizes foods with a low calorie density, which can increase weight loss and improve overall diet quality. However, it restricts some healthy food groups and is time-intensive.

It prioritizes low calorie, nutrient-dense foods with a high water content, which is thought to help keep you feeling full to encourage weight loss.

It categorizes foods based on their calorie density, prioritizing those that score very low. It also encourages you to get regular exercise, as well as log your food intake and physical activity and encourages regular exercise and emphasizes foods with a low calorie density, which are effective strategies to increase weight loss and reduce hunger and cravings.

The Volumetric Diet limits processed foods and may improve diet quality. It's also flexible and designed to be maintained long term.

The Volumetric Diet is time-intensive, and online resources are somewhat limited. It also restricts foods high in healthy fats, including nuts, seeds, and oils.

Foods with a very low calorie density include non-starchy veggies, broth-based soups, and fruits. These should comprise the bulk of your diet. Meanwhile, you should limit your intake of processed foods, nuts, seeds, and oils.

The meal plan above provides some simple meal and snack ideas for the Volumetric Diet.

Chapter one

The Volumetric Diet is an eating plan designed to promote weight loss by having you fill up on low calorie, nutrient-dense foods.

It's meant to reduce feelings of hunger by prioritizing foods with a high water content and low calorie density. It also encourages other healthy habits, such as regular exercise and keeping a food journal.

Still, you may wonder whether it's a good fit for you.

What is the Volumetric Diet?

The Volumetric Diet claims to help you feel full while eating fewer calories.

It's based on a book by nutrition scientist Dr. Barbara Rolls, which provides in-depth guidelines, recipes, and information on how to calculate the calorie density of your favorite foods.

The diet encourages you to eat nutrient-dense foods that are low in calories and high in water, such as fruits, vegetables, and soups. Meanwhile, it limits calorie-dense foods like cookies, candies, nuts, seeds, and oils.

Dr. Rolls asserts that these restrictions help you feel fuller for longer, cut your calorie intake, and promote weight loss.

Unlike other diets, the Volumetric Diet is intended to foster healthy eating habits and should be viewed as a long-term lifestyle change rather than a short-term solution.

How it works

The Volumetric Diet groups foods into four categories based on their calorie density:

Category 1 (very low calorie density): calorie density of less than 0.6

Category 2 (low calorie density): calorie density of 0.6–1.5

Category 3 (medium calorie density): calorie density of 1.6–3.9

Category 4 (high calorie density): calorie density of 4.0–9.0

Dr. Roll's book provides detailed information on how to calculate calorie density. In general, you should divide the number of calories in a particular serving size by its weight in grams. You'll end up with a figure between 0 and 9.

Foods with a high water content, such as broccoli, typically score very low in calorie density, while desserts and processed foods like dark chocolate usually rank high.

A typical meal on the Volumetric Diet should mostly comprise foods from Category 1, as well as include foods from Category 2 to help round out your plate. You can eat small amounts of foods from Category 3 and very limited portions from Category 4.

The diet's standard meal plan provides around 1,400 calories per day but can be adjusted to fit your calorie goals by adding extra snacks or increasing portion sizes.

No foods are completely off-limits on the Volumetric Diet. In fact, you can include foods with a high calorie density by modifying your portion sizes and adjusting your other meals.

Furthermore, the diet encourages at least 30–60 minutes of exercise each day.

You should keep track of your physical activity and food intake in a journal to monitor your progress and identify areas that may need improvement.

Does it work for weight loss?

Although few studies have examined the Volumetric Diet specifically, research suggests that its central tenets aid weight loss.

Promotes low calorie intake

Selecting foods with a low calorie density is particularly effective. Because these foods have a substantial volume but are low in calories, you can eat large servings without significantly increasing your calorie intake.

Notably, a review of 13 studies in 3,628 people tied foods with a lower calorie density to increased weight loss. Similarly, an 8-year study in over 50,000 women associated high-calorie-density foods with increased weight gain.

Choosing foods with a low calorie density may also help curb cravings and reduce appetite, which could boost weight loss.

A 12-week study in 96 women with excess weight and obesity found that meals with a lower calorie density led to decreased cravings, increased feelings of fullness, and reduced hunger.

In an older study in 39 women, participants ate 56% more calories when served a large portion of a high-calorie-density meal, compared with a smaller, low-calorie-density meal.

Encourages regular exercise

Exercise is another important component of the Volumetric Diet.

The diet recommends getting at least 30–60 minutes of physical activity per day, which may increase weight loss and fat loss by raising your energy expenditure, or the number of calories burned during the day.

Other health benefits

The Volumetric Diet may offer several other health benefits.

May boost diet quality

By encouraging healthy foods that are low in calories but high in fiber, vitamins, and minerals, the Volumetric Diet may help increase your intake of key nutrients and protect against nutritional deficiencies.

What's more, some research links diets with a low calorie density to improved diet quality.

Limits processed foods

Although the Volumetric Diet doesn't completely ban any foods, most processed foods have a high calorie density and should be restricted as part of the plan.

Processed foods are not only typically lacking in essential nutrients like fiber, protein, vitamins, and minerals but also usually higher in calories, fat, sugar, and sodium.

Furthermore, studies tie regular intake of processed foods to a higher risk of cancer, heart disease, and premature death.

Flexible and sustainable

Unlike most fad diets, the Volumetric Diet should be viewed as a long-term lifestyle change.

It pushes you to become more aware of your eating habits and food choices, which can help you make healthier dietary decisions by prioritizing foods with a lower calorie density, such as fruits and vegetables.

Additionally, because no foods are banned on the diet, you can enjoy your favorite dishes by making modifications and adjustments to your diet.

This may make the Volumetric Diet a good fit for people seeking some flexibility and a sustainable eating plan to follow long term.

Potential downsides

The Volumetric Diet has a few drawbacks to be aware of.

Time-intensive with few online resources

The diet requires significant time and energy investments, which may make it untenable for some people.

In addition to finding recipes, planning meals, and calculating calorie density, you're supposed to prepare most of your meals and snacks at home. This may make the diet too restrictive for those with a busy lifestyle, cramped kitchen, or limited access to fresh produce.

Although some support groups and recipes are available, online apps and resources for the diet are somewhat limited.

In fact, you may need to purchase the book by Dr. Rolls to calculate your meals' calorie density and track your food intake effectively.

Limits healthy fats

The diet also restricts certain foods rich in healthy fats, including nuts, seeds, and oils.

These foods provide monounsaturated and polyunsaturated fats, which may reduce inflammation and safeguard against chronic conditions like heart disease.

Moreover, many nutritious eating patterns like the Mediterranean diet encourage you to eat these foods.

Places too much emphasis on calories

Given that the Volumetric Diet is based on calorie density, high calorie foods are limited.

This means that nutritious, high calorie foods like avocados, nut butter, and whole eggs are limited, while processed, low calorie foods like fat-free salad dressing and diet ice cream are allowed due to their low calorie density.

Low calorie foods are often packed with added sugar and other unhealthy ingredients to enhance their taste. Just because something is low in calories doesn't mean it's healthy.

Foods to eat and avoid

Rather than banning any foods entirely, the Volumetric Diet divides them into four categories based on their calorie density.

Category 1

Foods in Category 1 have a very low calorie density and should comprise the majority of your diet. They include:

Fruits: apples, oranges, pears, peaches, bananas, berries, and grapefruit

Non-starchy vegetables: broccoli, cauliflower, carrots, tomatoes, zucchini, and kale

Soups: broth-based soups like vegetable soup, chicken soup, minestrone, and lentil soup

Nonfat dairy: skim milk and nonfat yogurt

Beverages: water, black coffee, and unsweetened tea

Category 2

Foods in the second category have a low energy density and can be enjoyed in moderation. They include:

Whole grains: quinoa, couscous, farro, buckwheat, barley, and brown rice

Legumes: chickpeas, lentils, black beans, and kidney beans

Starchy vegetables: potatoes, corn, peas, squash, and parsnips

Lean proteins: skinless poultry, white fish, and lean cuts of beef or pork

Category 3

Foods in the third category are considered medium calorie density. While they're permitted, it's important to keep an eye on serving sizes. These foods include:

Meat: fatty fish, poultry with the skin, and high fat cuts of pork and beef

Refined carbs: white bread, white rice, crackers, and white pasta

Full fat dairy: whole milk, full fat yogurt, ice cream, and cheese

Category 4

Foods in the final category are classified as high energy density. These foods contain lots of calories per serving and should be eaten sparingly. They include:

Nuts: almonds, walnuts, macadamia nuts, pecans, and pistachios

Seeds: chia seeds, sesame seeds, hemp seeds, and flax seeds

Oils: butter, vegetable oil, olive oil, margarine, and lard

Processed foods: cookies, candies, chips, pretzels, and fast food

Sample 3-day meal plan

On the Volumetric Diet, you should eat 3 meals per day, plus 2–3 snacks. Here's a 3-day sample menu:

Day 1

Breakfast: oatmeal with fruit and a glass of skim milk

Snack: carrots with hummus

Lunch: grilled chicken with quinoa and asparagus

Snack: sliced apples and light string cheese

Dinner: baked cod with spiced vegetable couscous

Breakfast: nonfat yogurt with strawberries and blueberries

Snack: a hard-boiled egg with tomato slices

Lunch: turkey chili with kidney beans and vegetables

Snack: a fruit salad with melon, kiwi, and strawberries

Dinner: zucchini boats stuffed with ground beef, tomatoes, bell peppers, and marinara sauce

Breakfast: scrambled eggs with mushrooms, tomatoes, and onions, plus a slice of whole wheat toast

Snack: a smoothie with skim milk, banana, and berries

Lunch: chicken noodle soup with a side salad

Snack: air-popped popcorn

Dinner: whole grain pasta with turkey meatballs and sautéed vegetables

What are the pros and cons of the volumetric diet?

Now, if alarm bells are ringing in your head, you're not alone. As we've written about before, not all high-calorie foods are "bad" for you. In fact, plenty of foods that are high in calories and fat are essential for good health, such as nuts, seeds, avocado, and fatty fish.

Pros:

This plan is it doesn't focus as much on what you can't eat, but rather what you can eat and how to portion out different kinds of food.

The diet allows for easy swaps. You could still eat a bowl of pasta on the volumetric diet, but instead of eating a whole bowl of pasta with just plain tomato sauce, you would swap half the pasta for veggies, like broccoli or mushrooms. "This way you are able to fill up on nutrient-rich foods that contain fewer calories rather than fill up solely on the pasta."

Unlike other plans that are low-carb and, in turn, can also be low fiber, the volumetric plan encourages fiber-rich foods, which can fill us up and keep us fuller longer on fewer calories. "It's a great way to keep you satiated and help you meet your daily nutrient goals.

Cons:

One potential drawback to this diet is that it recommends a very low consumption of nuts and seeds (since they are calorically dense). "Nuts and seeds provide monounsaturated fats and omega-3 fatty acids, both beneficial for cardiovascular and cognitive health."

Like many diet plans, it can also be difficult to dine out on the volumetric diet, since so many restaurants and food services prepare their food with high-calorie, high-fat butters and oils, Davis points out.

There is a volumetric book series on this diet that focuses on nutrition density and energy density. According to the books, foods with low energy density have few calorie contents, whereas foods with high density contain higher calories in each portion. And it also says that food items that are nutrient-dense have higher nutrient content compared to calories, and most of the time, they don't contain any added sugars, sodium, or saturated fat.

Basically, the volumetric diet is a specific strategy of eating habits that emphasize consuming high nutrition-dense foods such as vegetables, whole grains, low-fat dairy and fruits, and low energy-dense foods.

Benefits of Volumetric Diet

1. Sustainable Food Habits

The volumetric dieting plan has science backing its strategy, and that is why the plan has several health benefits. This diet is more about sustainable and healthy food habits rather than any food restriction.

2. Helps with Cardiovascular Diseases

Research suggests that the volumetric diet can help them in cardiovascular diseases as a low energy density diet contains fewer calories.

Type 2 diabetes, as the food items mentioned in the volumetric diet, does not contain any processed sugar or excessive glucose that can have the potential to increase the blood sugar level. Consuming low energy density food can help prevent post-menopause breast cancer.

3. Assists in Weight Loss

It is also one of the best diets for weight loss. According to several scientific research, it has been suggested that maintaining a healthy food diet without any additives and processed sugar, also consuming lower amounts of energy-dense food can help maintain the proper body weight, eliminating the excess fat buildup.

The ultimate volumetric diet plan is consuming food items mentioned in groups 1 and 2 for substance and energy, whereas keeping aside the food items mentioned in groups 3 and 4 for cheat days, once a week.

4. Volumetric Diet plan

The volumetric diets focus on what kind of foods to consume rather than eliminating certain groups of food items. The psychology of this diet is more about what should be consumed.

This diet divides food into 4 groups of diet plan and proportion control

Group 1:

The food items included in this group are non-starchy vegetables and fruits, along with nonfat dairy and thin broth-based soup.

Group 2: The food items included in this group are whole grains, low-fat meat, low-fat mixed dishes, breakfast cereal, starchy vegetables, and fruits.

Group 3: The food items included in this group are Pizza, cheese, meat, salad dressing, pretzels, bread, ice cream, cake, and several other similar food items.

Group 4: The food items included in this group are chips, crackers, chocolates, candies, oil, butter, nuts, and cookies

These are specific group portions. Group 1 is considered foods of high nutrient and low energy density. So low calories and are free to be consumed at all times. Whereas, the food energy density increases are of groups 2, 3, & 4. So the portion size should be controlled while consuming these groups of foods to avoid excessive energy intake.

The portion division isn't similar for everyone; it depends on individuals, muscle density, and body weight. Along with this, the volumetric diet also suggests exercising 30 minutes every day to eliminate any energy intake due to the consumption of food items mentioned in groups 2, 3, and 4.

What Foods Can Be Eaten and What Foods to Avoid?

Volumetric diet plan is really a strategy or meal plan that you should opt to stay healthy. A diet does not entirely restrict you from consuming any food group but teaches you how to consume all the foods you want and also maintain good health.

But there are certain suggestions in the volumetric diet books, such as it recommends food items with high water content and low energy density, high nutrient density, and high fiber. Food items such as fresh fruits (Refrain from consuming fruit juice or dried fruit), low-fat dairy, frozen, or fresh vegetables are helpful.

Additionally, food items such as pasta, legumes, beans, fiber-rich breakfast cereal, low-fat fish, lean meat, poultry without skin or fat, and whole grains are also beneficial. You can consume food items, such as low-fat yogurt, roasted or grilled meat, steamed veggies, grilled fish, and quinoa in larger quantities while following the volumetric diet plan.

Although this diet plan does not restrict any food item, it obviously mentions the proportion, decreasing, especially the food items mentioned in groups 3 and 4, as they have high energy density and low nutrient density. It also mentions to avoid any processed food items and stick to cooking food at home with fresh fruits and vegetables.

Risks and Side Effects

Even though the volumetric diet is quite helpful, it still has certain drawbacks. It mentions the low consumption of seeds and nuts as they are energy-dense. But research suggests that the human body gains Omega 3 fatty acids and monounsaturated fat from both nuts and seeds, which is beneficial for cognitive health and cardiovascular issues.

The volumetric diet does not exactly have a meal plan for any rigid restriction, which, even though is a good thing, can become a problem for people trying to follow a strict diet plan. Also, the low-density food with high water content keeps you full for the time being, not for a long period of time compared to the higher density foods.

Chapter two

Recipes

Peanut Butter Banana Chia Oatmeal

Prep Time: 5 minutes

Cook Time: 10 minutes

Total Time: 15 minutes

Yield: 2

INGREDIENTS

1 cup old fashioned oats

1 banana, sliced (save a few for topping)

1 Tablespoon chia seeds

1 teaspoon cinnamon

Pinch of sea salt

3 cups of water, non-dairy milk or a blend of both

2 Tablespoons peanut butter or another type of nut butter

Add oats, banana slices, chia seeds, cinnamon and sea salt to a pot. Add water and stir to combine. Heat over medium-high heat for 8-10 minutes or until all the liquid has been absorbed. Be sure to stir the oats several times while cooking to make sure the banana slices melt into the oats and the chia seeds don't clump. You'll know the oatmeal is done when all the liquid is absorbed and the oats are thick and fluffy.

Portion oats into two bowls and serve with peanut butter, banana slices, and a sprinkle of chia seeds. Add a splash of non-dairy milk and/or maple syrup on top before serving, if desired.

NUTRITION

Serving Size: 1 bowl

Calories: 369

Sugar: 10g

Fat: 12g

Carbohydrates: 61g

Fiber: 17g

Protein: 11g

Zucchini Noodle Pad Thai

Prep Time: 10 minutes

Cook Time: 15 minutes

Total Time: 25 minutes

Yield: 2

INGREDIENTS

1 teaspoon coconut oil

2 medium sized zucchinis, spiralized into noodles

2 cloves of garlic, minced

1 1/2 Tablespoons fresh ginger root, minced

1/2 cup red onion, chopped

1 carrot, spiralized or sliced into small strips using a vegetable peeler

1/2 red bell pepper, chopped

1 cup shelled edamame, cooked

2 Tablespoons natural creamy peanut butter

1/2 of a lime, juiced

1–2 Tablespoons water (for thinning out sauce)

1 teaspoon spicy chili paste like Sambal Oelek

Sea salt, to taste

1/4 cup fresh basil, chopped

2 Tablespoons chopped peanuts

INSTRUCTIONS

In a large skillet, heat coconut oil and sauté the garlic, ginger and red onion. Once onion is translucent and fragrant, stir in the red bell pepper, carrot slices and cooked edamame. Cook for 2-3 minutes.

Add a pinch of sea salt to the mixture, then add the lime juice, peanut butter, chili paste and a little water to thin out the sauce.

Place the zucchini noodles into the skillet and stir them around quite a bit so that the sauce coats them. Cook in sauce for about 8-10 minutes.

Remove from heat, plate and top with fresh basil and chopped peanuts. Enjoy.

NUTRITION
Serving Size: 1/2 of recipe

Calories: 292

Sugar: 10g

Fat: 14g

Carbohydrates: 28g

Fiber: 6g

Protein: 15g

Cauliflower Tabbouleh

Prep Time: 20 minutes

Total Time: 20 minutes

Yield: 6

INGREDIENTS

1 medium-large head of cauliflower

1 cup fresh flat-leaf parsley leaves, chopped

½ cup packed fresh mint leaves, chopped

3 green onions, thinly sliced

1 cup cherry or grape tomatoes, quartered or halved (depending on size)

1 cup cucumber, peeled and chopped

1/2 cup kalamata olives, pitted and chopped

3 small cloves of garlic, minced

1/4 cup fresh lemon juice

1 teaspoon apple cider vinegar

3 tablespoons extra-virgin olive oil

1 teaspoon fresh grated turmeric (or 1/2 teaspoon ground turmeric)

1/2–1 teaspoon fine sea salt

¼ teaspoon black pepper

INSTRUCTIONS

Cut the cauliflower to remove the stem and then chop into pieces small enough to fit into your food processor.

Place the cauliflower in food processor and pulse until the cauliflower pieces turn into cauliflower rice. You may have to do this in batches, depending on how large your processor is. Remove cauliflower rice from the processor and place in a large bowl.

Add parsley, mint, green onion and garlic into food processor to chop more finely, if desired.

Add parsley, mint, green onion and garlic into the bowl with the cauliflower rice. Add the remaining ingredients and toss to mix. Taste and add more salt or pepper if necessary.

Serve chilled or at room temperature. Store covered in the fridge for up to one week.

NUTRITION
Serving Size: 1/6 of recipe

Calories: 199

Sugar: 4g

Sodium: 751mg

Fat: 17g

Saturated Fat: 1g

Unsaturated Fat: 7g

Trans Fat: 0g

Carbohydrates: 8g

Fiber: 4g

Protein: 3g

Cholesterol: 0mg

Ultimate Smoothie Bowl
Yield: 1

INGREDIENTS

1/2 frozen banana, chopped into chunks

1 scoop chocolate protein powder

1/2 cup frozen mixed berries

1/2 cup unsweetened almond milk

1 teaspoon almond butter or peanut butter

TOPPINGS

1/4 of banana, sliced

1/4 cup fresh berries (I used strawberries and blueberries)

1 Tablespoon granola

1 teaspoon almond butter or peanut butter

1 teaspoon chia seeds

INSTRUCTIONS

Blend all the smoothie ingredients together in a high powdered blender until smooth. Pour into a bowl and top with toppings. Enjoy!

NUTRITION

Serving Size: 1

Calories: 343

Sugar: 21g

Fat: 12g

Carbohydrates: 48g

Fiber: 12g

Protein: 17g

Healthy Cauliflower Popcorn / Kettle Corn

Cook Time: 30 mins

Total Time: 30 mins

Yield: 2

INGREDIENTS

1 small/medium head cauliflower, cut into small florets (about 8 cups)

1 Tablespoon coconut oil, liquid

1 Tablespoon maple syrup

1/2 teaspoon sea salt

Heat oven to 425° F.

In a large bowl, stir together cauliflower, oil, maple syrup and 1/2 teaspoon salt.

Transfer to a baking sheet and spread in a single layer. Make sure the cauliflower pieces aren't too crowded on the baking sheet or they will steam instead of roasting.

Roast, stirring twice, until golden brown and tender, about 30 minutes. Serve hot.

Butternut Squash Fries

Prep Time: 10 minutes

Cook Time: 40 minutes

Total Time: 50 minutes

Yield: 4

INGREDIENTS

1 butternut squash (about 4 cups)

Sea salt

INSTRUCTIONS

Pre-heat oven to 425°F.

Peel the squash. (Optional)

Cut the butternut squash in half and de-seed it like you would a cantaloupe.

Cut it up into French fry shapes. Try to make the pieces similar in size so that they finish cooking at the same time.

Place on a baking sheet lined with parchment paper or sprayed with nonstick cooking spray. Sprinkle lightly with sea salt.

Place tray in your pre-heated oven and bake for 40 minutes or so, flipping halfway through baking process.

Fries are done when they are starting to brown a little.

Serve with ketchup or your favorite French fry dipping sauce.

Serving Size: 1 cup

Calories: 63

Sugar: 3g

Fat: 0g

Carbohydrates: 16g

Fiber: 3g

Protein: 1g

Mixed Berry Fruit Salad
Yield: 4

1 lb. quartered strawberries

1 pint blueberries

2 cups fresh pineapple chunks

3 kiwi, peeled, halved and sliced

2 cups seedless grapes

2 tablespoons lime juice

1/4 teaspoon grated lime zest

1 tablespoon maple syrup

1/2 teaspoon poppy seeds

INSTRUCTIONS

In a large bowl toss together strawberries, blueberries, pineapple, kiwi and grapes. In a small bowl, whisk together lime juice, lime zest, maple syrup and poppy seeds. Drizzle lime dressing over fresh fruit mixture, toss and serve immediately.

NUTRITION

Serving Size: 1/4 of recipe

Calories: 200

Sugar: 38g

Fat: 1g

Carbohydrates: 48g

Fiber: 7g

Protein: 3g

Zucchini Noodle Fettuccine With Cauliflower Alfredo

Yield: 2

INGREDIENTS

2 cups steamed cauliflower, divided 1 1/2 cups for sauce, 1/2 cup for pasta dish

1/4–1/3 cup unsweetened original Almond Breeze almond milk

2 cloves roasted garlic

1 Tablespoon nutritional yeast

1/2–1 Tablespoon olive or avocado oil

1/2 teaspoon sea salt

1/4 teaspoon ground pepper

1/4 cup red onion, chopped

4 baby bella mushrooms, sliced

2 medium-large zucchini squash

Fresh basil and chopped red onion (optional for serving)

Steam cauliflower if you haven't already.

While cauliflower is steaming, make fettuccine noodles by spiralizing your zucchini using the correct blade. Set noodles aside.

Prepare cauliflower Alfredo sauce but placing 1 1/2 cups steamed cauliflower, almond milk, roasted garlic, nutritional yeast, oil, salt and pepper into a blender. Blend until smooth. You want the sauce to be kind of thick (like regular Alfredo sauce) but not too thick so add a bit more almond milk if needed. Set aside.

In a extra-large skillet over medium heat, add a little oil, onions and mushrooms. Sauté for 3-5 minutes or until onions are fragrant and mushrooms has softened. Add zucchini noodles to the pan and cook until noodles are hot and al dente, about 3-5 minutes more. Drain any excess liquid from the pan if needed. Add cauliflower sauce and remaining cauliflower florets to pan and mix well to combine. Toss well until all noodles are coated with sauce. Heat until pasta is warm and ready to serve.

Serve with a sprinkle of extra chopped onion. Season with salt and pepper to taste.

Serving Size: 1/2 recipe

Calories: 169

Sugar: 8g

Fat: 6g

Carbohydrates: 23g

Fiber: 8g

Protein: 10g

Stuffed Spaghetti Squash Lasagna Bowls

Prep Time: 10 minutes

Cook Time: 60 minutes

Total Time: 1 hour 10 minutes

Yield: 2

INGREDIENTS

1 spaghetti squash

1 cup marinara sauce

1/2 cup vegan ricotta cheese* (I used Kite Hill)

1/2 cup baby greens (spinach or arugula work great)

Crumbled vegan ricotta cheese, for topping

Hemp parmesan, for topping

INSTRUCTIONS

Heat oven to 350°F. Chop spaghetti squash in half length wise, scoop out seeds with a spoon. Coat the inside of each half with a little olive oil, salt and pepper. Place on a baking sheet, cut side down and bake for about 40-50 minutes or until you can easily pierce a fork through the squash. Let stand for 10 minutes, scrape the inside of the squash with a fork to remove the spaghetti-like strands.

Combine spaghetti squash strands, marinara sauce, ricotta cheese and baby greens in a bowl.

Increase oven to temperature to broil.

Spoon spaghetti squash mixture into the bottom of each squash half. Top with a little crumbed ricotta cheese and broil for about 5-7 minutes or until ricotta gets a little golden.

Remove from oven, sprinkle with a little hemp parmesan and enjoy!

NUTRITION

Serving Size: 1/2 squash w/o hemp parm

Calories: 318

Sugar: 6g

Fat: 20g

Carbohydrates: 27g

Fiber: 5g

Protein: 12g

Healthy Chocolate Banana Ice Cream

Prep Time: 10 minutes

Total Time: 10 minutes

Yield: 2 servings

INGREDIENTS

3 frozen bananas, chopped into chunks

1/4 cup almond milk (unsweetened chocolate or vanilla)

1 Tablespoon almond butter

1/2 – 1 Tablespoon cacao powder (or cocoa powder)

1/2 Tablespoons cacao nibs or chocolate chips (optional)

INSTRUCTIONS

Place bananas, almond milk, almond butter and cocoa powder into a food processor or high speed blender.

Pulse/process until smooth and creamy. You may need to turn off the motor and stir the mixture a couple times while processing.

Add in cacao nibs or chocolate chips (if using) and pulse once more. Spoon ice cream in to a bowl and enjoy! If you want to be able to scoop the ice cream you can place it in the freezer for 2 hours so it's solid enough to scoop.

Serving Size: 1/2 of recipe

Calories: 240

Sugar: 23g

Sodium: 26mg

Fat: 7g

Saturated Fat: 2g

Unsaturated Fat: 0g

Trans Fat: 0g

Carbohydrates: 47g

Fiber: 7g

Protein: 4g

Cholesterol: 0mg

Tofu Veggie Noodle Bowl With Cabbage Noodles

Prep Time: 20 mins

Cook Time: 10 mins

Total Time: 30 mins

Yield: 3

INGREDIENTS

12 ounces extra firm tofu, pressed and drained

½ cup vegetable stock

1 Tablespoon low sodium tamari

½ teaspoon maple syrup

1 Tablespoon rice wine vinegar

1 teaspoon sesame oil

1 ½ Tablespoons coconut oil

1 Tablespoon minced ginger

1 Tablespoons minced garlic (2–3 large cloves)

1–2 cups fresh broccoli, chopped into bite-size florets

1 medium cabbage, thinly sliced (about 1/2 pound, 5 cups chopped)

1 green pepper, cut into thin strips

2 carrots, peeled and cut into thin strips

¼ cup roughly chopped walnuts

sea salt, to taste

Fresh ground pepper, to taste

Cut the tofu into small cubes.

In a small bowl combine the vegetable stock, tamari, maple syrup, rice wine vinegar and sesame oil. Set aside.

Heat a large wok or skillet over high heat. Add in 1 tablespoon of coconut oil. Once melted, add the tofu and stir-fry until golden, about 3 minutes. Transfer to a plate.

Add the remaining coconut oil into the same skillet. Add the garlic and ginger and stir-fry for about 30 seconds, until fragrant. Add the bell pepper, carrot and broccoli and stir-fry for 1 minute, or until they begin to soften. Then add the cabbage. Stir-fry for 1 minute, add salt and pepper to taste, and stir-fry for another 1-2 minutes.

Return the tofu to the skillet, stir in the walnuts and the stock/soy sauce mixture and stir-fry for another minute, until it has just about evaporated. It's okay if there's still a little liquid in the pan. Remove from the heat and serve.

Serving Size: 1/3 of recipe

Calories: 344

Sugar: 12g

Fat: 21g

Carbohydrates: 26g

Fiber: 9g

Protein: 17g

Chapter three

Conclusion

The Volumetric diet is one of the best-known weight loss programs as it helps eliminate all processed foods from your general diet. It suggests mainly to consume organic and whole foods that are good for the body.

But it's necessary to consult a dietician or a nutritionist before following the volumetric diet so that you can get the actual food items that you should and shouldn't eat during the diet along with their proportions. Volumetric diet is one of the top weight loss diets as it regularly maintains the calorie intake and general food consumption is very calculated.

The Volumetric Diet prioritizes foods with a low calorie density and high volume. It promotes weight loss by enhancing feelings of fullness while reducing hunger and cravings.

It may also improve your diet quality by increasing your intake of nutrient-dense foods like fruits and vegetables.

However, the Volumetric Diet also requires substantial time and energy, restricts several healthy foods, and offers limited online resources, which may make it unsuitable for some people.

If the thought of prepping and eating more low-density foods, skipping calorie counts, and simply moving around more sounds doable, you may be the perfect candidate to give the Volumetric diet a try.

Made in the USA
Middletown, DE
18 July 2023

35411456R00040